Chronic Lymphocytic Leukemia (CLL): Fast Focus Study Guide

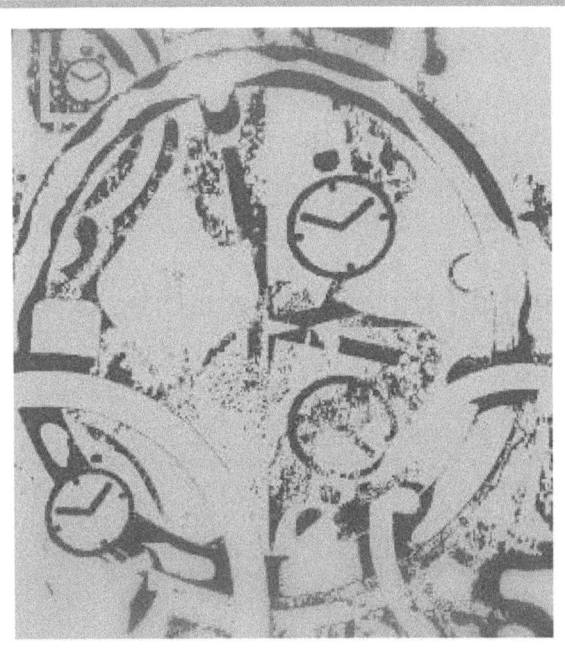

Acknowledgements

I dedicate this book to my beautiful
wife and children, who I love more
than all the water in all the oceans
and all the seas.

CONTENTS

- This book is written for medical students, residents, and physicians who want to learn more about chronic lymphocytic leukemia.

- Put this book in your bathroom or on your coffee table.

- This is a great resource for any medical professional.

- This Fast Focus Study Guide will provide you with a practical review of the key information you need to know.

- Buy this book now if you want this quick and concise information

CLL is a leukemia characterized by the proliferation and accumulation of small mature lymphocytes within the blood, bone marrow, lymph nodes, and spleen.

Chronic lymphocytic leukemia (CLL) is the most common type of leukemia in Western countries and has an incidence of 4.3/ 100,000 people in the United States.

The diagnosis of chronic lymphocytic leukemia is usually suspected when a patients present with an elevated white blood cell count on CBC associated with a relative lymphocytosis on differential. Often characteristic smudge cells are seen. The diagnosis is confirmed by sending peripheral blood for flow cytometry.

If the number of lymphocytes is < 5 x 109/L cells then the patient does not meet the criteria of CLL. This condition is called a monoclonal B-cell lymphocytosis.

The median age at CLL diagnosis is between 67 and 72 years. More male than female patients are affected by this disease.

Only 10% of patients diagnosed with CLL are younger than 50 years old.

About 10% of people diagnosed with CLL
have a first-generation relative with CLL.

People diagnosed with CLL often are at increased risk of infection. Hypogammaglobulinemia is seen in about 25% of cases and is characterized with depressed levels of IgG, IgA, or IgM.

The most common infections in patients with hypogammaglobulinemia occur in the respiratory tract and are caused by encapsulated organisms such as Steptococcus pneumoniae and Haemophilus influenzae.

Treating the CLL can improve hypogammagloblulinemia but sometimes treatment with intravenous pooled human immunoglobulin is required.

Autoimmune disorders such as autoimmune hemolytic anemia (AIHA) and autoimmune thrombocytopenic purpura (ITP). Other autoimmune disorders such as pure red cell aplasia, neutropenia, and angioedema can also manifest in patients with CLL.

At the time of initial diagnosis patients should undergo flow cytometry to confirm the diagnosis. Additional testing should include interphase cytogenetics and VH gene status assessment. The ZAP-70 expression by flow cytometry is typically not recommended. CT scans are not needed unless there are symptoms. PET scan can be helpful if Richter's suspected. Bone marrow aspirate and biopsy are not needed unless there is evidence of low blood counts that need additional evaluation.

Small lymphocytic lymphoma (SLL) has the same biology and clinical features as CLL however SLL is characterized by lymphadenopathy and bone marrow involvement without elevated abnormal cells in the peripheral blood.

The overall median survival of all patients with CLL is approximately nine years.

There are many ways to further characterize the prognosis in patients with CLL to determine when and how to treat the disease.

High serum levels of beta 2 microglobulin and insoluble CD23 are poor prognostic factors in patients with chronic lymphocytic leukemia.

The Zap-70 mutation in patients with chronic lymphocytic leukemia is associated with a worse prognosis characterized by early progression and decreased survival.

CD38 corresponds to the un-mutated, naïve B-cell chronic lymphocytic leukemia. We know that these patients are known to have a worse prognosis.

Cytogenetics are commonly used to differentiate patients with a poor prognosis.

All patients with CLL should have blood sent for interphase cytogenetics looking for +12, del(13q), del(17)(p13.1) and del(11)(q22.3).

Patients with chromosome 17p have the worst prognosis. 11q deletions are not as bad but are also refractory to chemotherapy and have a poor prognosis.

Patients 13q deletions are associated with a better prognosis in patients with CLL.

CLL Cytogenetics

del(17)(p13.1)

% of patients- 7%

Median time to treatment- 9 months

Median overall survival- 22 months

CLL Cytogenetics

Trisomy 12

% of patients- 14%

Median time to treatment- 33 months

Median overall survival- 114 months

CLL Cytogenetics

del(13)(q14)

% of patients- 55%

Median time to treatment- 49 months

Median overall survival- 133 months

CLL Cytogenetics

None detected

% of patients- 18%

Median time to treatment- 92 months

Median overall survival- 111 months

The Rai Staging System is outlined on the
following pages.

Stage 0 CLL is characterized by lymphocytosis only.

Stage I chronic lymphocytic leukemia is characterized by lymphadenopathy.

Stage II chronic lymphocytic leukemia is

characterized by hepatosplenomegaly.

Stage III chronic lymphocytic leukemia is characterized by anemia.

Stage IV chronic lymphocytic leukemia is characterized by thrombocytopenia.

The doubling time and the total white blood count are not indications to treat CLL as long as the lymphocyte count is <300,000 cells/μL.

Cytogenetics alone are generally not
considered a reason to treat.

If the lymphocyte count is < 300,000 then we treat if symptoms develop. We would treat if the patient has enlarging, symptomatic lymph nodes; enlarging, symptomatic spleen; cytopenias due to CLL (hemoglobin < 11 g/dL, platelets < 100,000 cells/µL); constitutional symptoms due to disease such as fatigue and B symptoms; or poorly controlled AIHA or ITP.

There are many old and new treatment options available for CLL.

Monotherapy with alkylating agents such as chorambucil has been a first line therapy for CLL for a long time.

Bendamustine was superior when it was compared with chlorambucil in a randomized trial. Bendamustine produced improved responses but greater toxicity and no OS benefit. The overall response rate (ORR) was 67% versus 30% and the median progression-free survival (PFS) was 22 months versus 8 months.

Bendamustine has been combined with rituximab in patients with relapsed CLL. Patients received 70 mg/m2 of bendamustine on days 1 and 2 and 375 mg/m2 of rituximab on day 0 of the first cycle and 500 mg/m2 on day 1 of subsequent cycles administered every 28 days for up to 6 cycles. The ORR was 59.0%. The ORR was 45.5 % in fludarabine-refractory patients and 60.5% in fludarabine-sensitive patients. After a median follow-up time of 24 months, the median event-free survival was 14.7 months.

When bendamustine was combined with
rituximab the overall response rate by genetic
subgroups indicated that 92.3% of patients
with del(11q), 100% with trisomy 12, 7.1%
with del(17p), and 58.7% with unmutated
IGHV status responded to treatment.

The dose-modified FCR-Lite regimen decreased the dose of fludarabine and cyclophosphamide, increased the dose of rituximab, and used a maintenance regimen for rituximab given every 3 months until progression. The CR rate was 77% for 50 previously untreated CLL patients with an ORR of 100%.

Alemtuzumab is a recombinant monoclonal antibody against the CD52 antigen. Monotherapy with alemtuzumab has produced response rates of 33% to 53%, with a median duration of response ranging from 8.7 to 15.4 months, in patients with advanced CLL who were previously treated with alkylating agents and had failed or relapsed after second-line fludarabine therapy.

Alemtuzumab has been proven effective in patients with high-risk genetic markers such as deletions of chromosome 11 or 17.

Ofatumumab is a fully humanized antibody targeting a unique epitope on the CD20 molecule expressed on human B cells. When used for the treatment of CLL refractory to fludarabine and alemtuzumab, the ORR was 58%. The ORR was 47% in the bulky disease group.

Obinutuzumab is a humanized monoclonal antibody that showed impressive results in vitro with higher rates of apoptosis in malignant B cells compared with rituximab. Phase I/II study in relapsed disease shows acceptable safety and ORR 20%.

Idelalisib is a PI3Ks inhibitor. In CLL, the PI3K pathway is constitutively activated and dependent on PI3Kδ. Idelasib is an oral PI3Kδ isoform–selective inhibitor that promotes apoptosis in primary CLL cells.

Ibrutinib is a BTK inhibitor that is orally active small molecule inhibiting BTK that can induce apoptosis in B-cell lymphomas and CLL cells.

As a general rule, the frontline treatment may be repeated if the duration of the first remission exceeds 24 months provided that the frontline therapy was well tolerated.

Data from a phase 1b-2 multicenter study with single-agent ibrutinib in patients with relapsed or refractory CLL or small lymphocytic lymphoma. The majority of whom had high-risk disease. The ORR was 71%, the majority being PRs (68%) and the response was independent of clinical and genomic risk factors, including advanced-stage disease, the number of previous therapies, and del(17p). At 26 months, the estimated PFS rate was 75% and the OS rate was 83%.

Ibrutinib on side effects were generally mild and included transient diarrhea, fatigue, and upper respiratory tract infection.

Lenalidomide has shown encouraging results in the treatment of high-risk patients, including carriers of a del(17p) and fludarabine refractory CLL. The ORR of lenalidomide monotherapy varied between 32% and 54% in different clinical trials.

Treatment with lenalidomide is associated with myelosuppression and a tumor flare reaction. The tumor flare is characterized by a marked and painful increase in lymph nodes size, malaise, and fever. The tumor flare reaction is more common in CLL than in other lymphoid malignancies.

Ablative stem cell transplants have a 40% to 50% 100-day mortality in CLL patients. The non-ablative approach using immunosuppressive therapy followed by administration of donor cells lowers year mortality to 10% to 20%. These patients have a 30% to 40% EFS at 4 years.

This concludes Porphyria: Fast Focus Study Guide

Search Amazon Kindle books to find other study guides written by

JT Thomas, MD

Internal Medicine Study Guide

Hematology Study Guide

Medical Oncology Study Guide

Rheumatology Study Guide

www.ingramcontent.com/pod-product-compliance
Lightning Source LLC
Chambersburg PA
CBHW071000180526
45168CB00003B/1224